DIABETIC COOKBOOK AND MEAL PREP FOR BEGINNERS

PREVENT AND REVERSE DIABETES TYPE 1 AND TYPE 2 WITH A FRIENDLY GUIDE TO LOSE WEIGHT AND BURN FAT WITH LOW BUDGET RECIPES. MANAGE QUICKLY AND EASILY DISEASE WITH HEALTHY, LOW CARB AND FULL PROOFED DELICIOUS RECIPES.

KAREN L. RAMOS

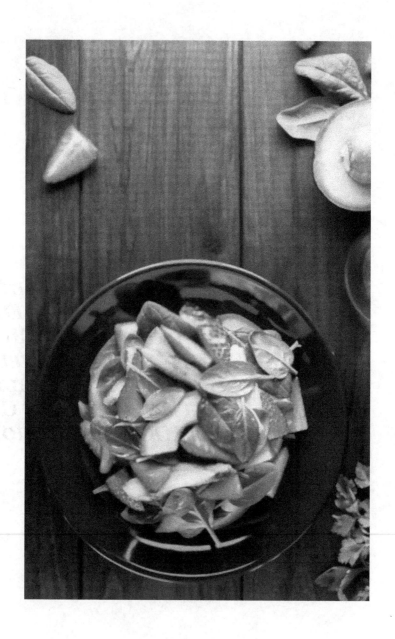

© Copyright 2021 by KAREN L. RAMOS All rights reserved. The following Book is reproduced below with the goal of providing information that is as accurate and reliable as possible. Regardless, purchasing this Book can be seen as consent to the fact that both the publisher and the author of this book are in no way experts on the topics discussed within and that any recommendations or suggestions that are made herein are for entertainment purposes only. Professionals should be consulted as needed prior to undertaking any of the action endorsed herein.

This declaration is deemed fair and valid by both the American Bar Association and the Committee of Publishers Association and is legally binding throughout the United States.

Furthermore, the transmission, duplication, or reproduction of any of the following work including specific information will be considered an illegal act irrespective of if it is done electronically or in print. This extends to creating a secondary or tertiary copy of the work or a recorded copy and is only allowed with the express written consent from the Publisher. All additional right reserved.

The information in the following pages is broadly considered a truthful and accurate account of facts and as such, any inattention, use, or misuse of the information in question by the reader will render any resulting actions solely under their purview. There are no scenarios in which the publisher or the original author of this work can be in any fashion deemed liable for any hardship or damages that may befall them after undertaking information described herein.

Additionally, the information in the following pages is intended only for informational purposes and should thus be thought of as universal. As befitting its nature, it is presented without assurance regarding its prolonged validity or interim quality. Trademarks that are mentioned are done without written consent and can in no way be considered an endorsement from the trademark holder.

Table Of Contents

DIABETIC COOKBOOK AND MEAL PREP FOR BEGINNERS 1

INTRODUCTION 10

BREAKFAST 16
- BUCKWHEAT PORRIDGE 16
- BREAKFAST SANDWICH 19
- BERRY-OAT BREAKFAST BARS 20
- EGGPLANT OMELET 23
- BREAKFAST MUFFINS 25

MEAT 27
- MEATBALLS IN TOMATO GRAVY 27
- GARLIC-BRAISED SHORT RIB 31
- PULLED PORK 33
- ROSEMARY-GARLIC LAMB RACKS 34
- IRISH PORK ROAST 36

FISH AND SEAFOOD 39
- HERBED SALMON 39
- SALMON IN GREEN SAUCE 41
- BRAISED SHRIMP 43
- SHRIMP COCONUT CURRY 45

DESSERTS 47
- RASPBERRY CAKE WITH WHITE CHOCOLATE SAUCE 47
- KETOGENIC LAVA CAKE 49
- KETOGENIC CHEESE CAKE 50
- CAKE WITH WHIPPED CREAM ICING 52
- WALNUT-FRUIT CAKE 54

MORE RECIPES 57
- TABBOULEH- ARABIAN SALAD 57
- CHEESE STUFF PEPPERS 59
- ROASTED PEPPER SALAD 60
- BREAKFAST CASSEROLE DELICIOUS 61
- HUEVOS RANCHEROS 62
- FLOURLESS BROCCOLI CHEESE QUICHE 64
- ASPARAGUS CHEESE STRATA 66
- ALMOND CRUNCH GRANOLA 68
- VEGETABLE FRITTATA 70
- BREAKFAST BURRITO 72
- PUMPKIN OATMEAL WITH RAISINS 74

Mushroom and Black Bean Burrito	75
Shrimp with Green Beans	77
Crab Curry	79
Mixed Chowder	80
Mussels in Tomato Sauce	81
Citrus Salmon	82
Pork with Bell Peppers	84
Roasted Pork Shoulder	86
Pork Chops in Peach Glaze	88
Ground Pork with Spinach	90
Yogurt Raspberry Cake	92
Turkey Egg Casserole	93
Mixed Berry Dutch Pancake	94
Jalapeño Potato Hash	96
Bacon and Egg Sandwiches	98
Spinach and Tomato Egg Cup	100
Egg Muffins with Bell Pepper	101
Tomato and Spinach Egg Cup	103
Egg and Cheese Pockets	104
Leftovers Bubble and Squeak	106
CONCLUSION	**108**

Introduction

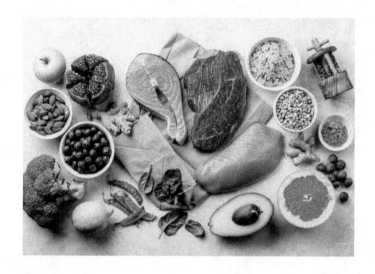

The Benefits of the Diabetes Meal Prep

Meal planning is extremely helpful in many practical ways, but one of its greatest benefits is on a person's health, particularly if it combines healthy balanced food and proper portion control.

Benefit # 1 - It helps improve your general health

Whether or not you have a medical condition, meal planning can help you improve your overall health when the meals provide all the macro and micronutrients your body needs. It also helps you avoid saturated fats and processed sugars, which is what most people would reach for if they're hungry and just want something satisfying.

Benefit # 2 - It ensures that you can eat on time

Preparing your meals in advance helps manage hunger pains. Missing a meal or delaying it can cause your blood sugar level to drop too low, a condition otherwise known as hypoglycemia.

Hypoglycemia can cause shaking, disorientation, and irritability. You may even have a seizure if your blood sugar level gets any lower. Having your meal already prepared ensures that you can always eat on time and, therefore, decrease the risk of low blood glucose.

Benefit # 3 - It lowers your risk of heart disease

Diabetes increases the risk of heart disease. With the help of a dietician, planning your meals can help you reduce this risk. Because meal prep reduces the time you need to spend in the kitchen, you'll have more opportunities to exercise and do other activities that promote a healthier lifestyle.

Benefit # 4 - It lowers your risk of cancer

Diabetes also increases the risk of all forms of cancer. While experts are still unable to identify the exact link between these two conditions, they expect that it has something to do with insulin resistance and obesity. Cancer patients are advised to pursue a healthy lifestyle, which includes eating a balanced diet and getting adequate exercise. Because these activities are also encouraged among diabetics, the risk of cancer is lowered.

Benefit # 5 - It helps you maintain healthy body weight

Again, portion control plays a part in this area. Even if you eat healthy food, overindulging can lead to an unhealthy weight gain, which can make it harder to control your blood sugar level.

If left unchecked, this could lead to high blood sugar levels or hyperglycemia, which can cause various complications that include heart and liver damage as well as the loss of kidney function.

It's important to note that while meal planning can help keep the effects of diabetes under control, you and your dietician still need to conduct a periodic review of its effectiveness and make changes whenever necessary.

How to identify if you have Diabetes

The early signs of diabetes include:

- Hunger and fatigue

When your body consumes food, it converts it into glucose so that the cells can use it for energy. The body needs insulin so that the cells can take in the glucose. Without enough insulin or if the cells are unable to use insulin, the body does not get any energy, making you feel tired as well as hungry all the time.

- Excessive thirst and urination

Usually, a person pees from four to seven times a day. But with people who suffer from diabetes pee a lot more. This also makes you thirsty more frequently.

- Dry mouth and itchy skin

When the body uses fluids to create urine, it has less moisture to keep the mouth and skin from drying.

- Blurry vision

Changes in the body's fluid levels can inflame the lens of the eyes, making it more difficult for the eyes to focus.

Symptoms of type-2 diabetes include:

- Yeast infections
- Slow-healing wounds
- Pain in the muscles
- Numbness of legs and feet

Symptoms of type-1 diabetes are the following:

- Unexplained weight loss
- Nausea and vomiting

As for gestational diabetes, there are no symptoms. The condition is only determined during prenatal screening.

Breakfast

Buckwheat Porridge

Servings: 2 Cooking Time: 15 Minutes

Ingredients:

- 1½ cups water
- cup buckwheat groats, rinsed
- ¾ teaspoon vanilla extract
- ½ teaspoon ground cinnamon
- ¼ teaspoon salt
- 2 tablespoons maple syrup
- ripe banana, peeled and mashed
- 1½ cups unsweetened soy milk
- tablespoon peanut butter
- 1/3 cup fresh strawberries, hulled and chopped

Direction:

- Place the water, buckwheat, vanilla extract, cinnamon, and salt in a pan and bring to a boil.
- Now, adjust the heat to medium-low and simmer for about 6 minutes, stirring occasionally.
- Stir in maple syrup, banana, and soy milk, and simmer,

covered for about 6 minutes.

- Remove the pan of porridge from heat and stir in peanut butter.
- Serve warm with the topping of strawberry pieces.

Nutrition: Calories 453 Total Fat 9.4 g Saturated Fat 1.7 g Cholesterol 0 mg Sodium 374 mg Total Carbs 82.8 g Fiber 9.4 g Sugar 28.8 g Protein 16.2 g

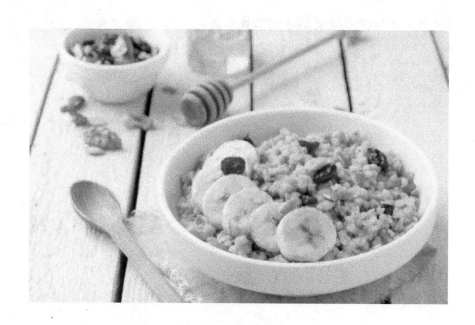

Breakfast Sandwich

Servings: 2 Cooking Time: 0 Minutes

Ingredients:

- 2 oz/60g cheddar cheese
- 1/6 oz/30g smoked ham
- 2 tbsp butter 4 eggs

Direction:

- Fry all the eggs and sprinkle the pepper and salt on them.
- Place an egg down as the sandwich base.
- Top with the ham and cheese and a drop or two of Tabasco.
- Place the other egg on top and enjoy.

Nutrition: 600 cal.50g fat 12g protein 7g carbs.

Berry-oat Breakfast Bars

Servings: 12 Cooking Time: 25 Minutes

Ingredients:

- 2 cups fresh raspberries or blueberries
- 2 tablespoons sugar
- 2 tablespoons freshly squeezed lemon juice
- 1 tablespoon cornstarch
- 1 1/2 cups rolled oats
- 1/2 cup whole-wheat flour
- 1/2 cup walnuts
- ¼ cup chia seeds
- ¼ cup extra-virgin olive oil
- ¼ cup honey
- large egg

Direction:

- Preheat the oven to 350F. In a small saucepan over medium heat, stir together the berries, sugar, lemon juice, and cornstarch.
- Bring to a simmer. Reduce the heat and simmer for 2 to 3 minutes, until the mixture thickens.
- In a food processor or high-speed blender, combine the oats,

flour, walnuts, and chia seeds.

- Process until powdered. Add the olive oil, honey, and egg.
- Pulse a few more times, until well combined. Press half of the mixture into a 9-inch square baking dish. Spread the berry filling over the oat mixture. Add the remaining oat mixture on top of the berries.
- Bake for 25 minutes, until browned. Let cool completely, cut into 12 pieces, and serve. Store in a covered container for up to 5 days.

Nutrition: Calories: 201; Total fat: 10g; Saturated fat: 1g; Protein: 5g; Carbs: 26g; Sugar: 9g; Fiber: 5g; Cholesterol: 16mg; Sodium: 8mg

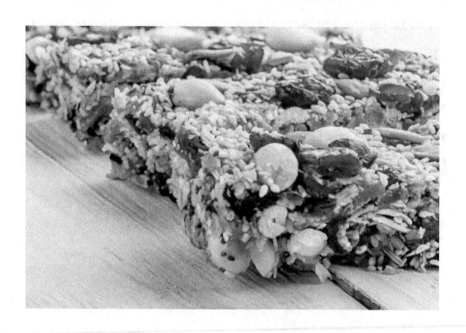

Eggplant Omelet

Servings: 2 Cooking Time: 5 Minutes

Ingredients:

- large eggplant
- 1 tbsp coconut oil, melted
- 1 tsp unsalted butter
- 2 eggs
- 2 tbsp chopped green onions

Direction:

- Set the grill and let it preheat at the high setting.
- In the meantime, prepare the eggplant, and for this, cut two slices from eggplant, about 1-inch thick, and reserve the remaining eggplant for later use.
- Brush slices of eggplant with oil, season with salt on both sides, then put the slices on grill and cook for 3 to 4 minutes per side.
- Move grilled eggplant to a cutting board, let it cool for 5 minutes and then make a home in the center of each slice by using a cookie cutter.
- Bring out a frying pan, put it over medium heat, add butter and when it melts, add eggplant slices in it and crack an egg into its each hole.

- Let the eggs cook, then carefully flip the eggplant slice and continue cooking for 3 minutes until the egg has thoroughly cooked Season egg with salt and black pepper, move them to a plate, then garnish with green onions and serve.

Nutrition:184 Cal 14.1 g Fats 7.8 g Protein 3 g Net Carb 3.5 g Fiber

Breakfast Muffins

Servings: 1 Cooking Time: 5 Minutes

Ingredients:

- medium egg
- ¼ cup heavy cream
- 1 slice cooked bacon (cured, pan-fried, cooked)
- 1 oz cheddar cheese
- Salt and black pepper (to taste)

Direction:

- Preheat the oven to 350°F.
- In a bowl, mix the eggs with the cream, salt and pepper.
- Spread into muffin tins and fill the cups half full.
- Place 1 slice of bacon into each muffin hole and half ounce of cheese on top of each muffin.
- Bake for around 15-20 minutes or until slightly browned.
- Add another ½ oz of cheese onto each muffin and broil until the cheese is slightly browned.
- Serve!

Nutrition: 150 cal 11g fat 7g protein 2g carbs

Meat

Meatballs In Tomato Gravy

Servings: 6 Cooking Time: 30 Minutes

Ingredients:

- For Meatballs:
- pound lean ground lamb
- tablespoon homemade tomato paste
- ¼ cup fresh cilantro leaves, chopped
- 1 small onion, chopped finely
- 2 garlic cloves, minced
- ½ teaspoon ground cumin
- 1/8 teaspoon salt Ground black pepper, as required
- For Tomato Gravy:
- 3 tablespoons olive oil, divided
- 2 medium onions, chopped finely
- 2 garlic cloves, minced
- ½ tablespoon fresh ginger, minced
- teaspoon dried thyme, crushed
- teaspoon dried oregano, crushed
- 3 large tomatoes, chopped finely Ground black pepper, as required

- 1½ cups warm low-sodium chicken broth

Direction:

- For meatballs: in a large bowl, add all the ingredients and mix until well combined. Make small equal-sized balls from mixture and set aside.
- For gravy: in a large pan, heat 1 tablespoon of oil over medium heat.
- Add the meatballs and cook for about 4-5 minutes or until lightly browned from all sides. With a slotted spoon, transfer the meatballs onto a plate.
- In the same pan, heat the remaining oil over medium heat and sauté the onion for about 8-10 minutes. Add the garlic, ginger and herbs and sauté for about 1 minute.   . Add the tomatoes and cook for about 3-4 minutes, crushing with the back of spoon. Add the warm broth and bring to a boil.
- Carefully, place the meatballs and cook for 5 minutes, without stirring.
- Now, reduce the heat to low and cook partially covered for about 15-20 minutes, stirring gently 2-3 times. Serve hot.
- Meal Prep Tip:
- Transfer the meatballs mixture into a large bowl and set aside to cool. Divide the mixture into 6 containers evenly. Cover the containers and refrigerate for 1-2 days.

- Reheat in the microwave before serving.

Nutrition: Calories 248 Total Fat 12.9 g Saturated Fat 3 g Cholesterol 68 mg Total Carbs 10 g Sugar 4.8 g Fiber 2.5 g Sodium 138 mg Potassium 591 mg Protein 23.4 g

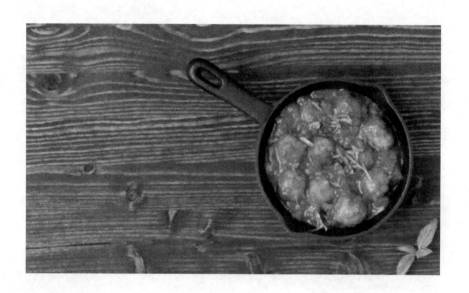

Garlic-braised Short Rib

Servings: 4 Cooking Time: 2 Hours, 20 Minutes

Ingredients:

- 4 (4-ounce) beef short ribs
- Sea salt
- Freshly ground black pepper
- 1 tablespoon olive oil
- 2 teaspoons minced garlic
- ½ cup dry red wine
- 3 cups Rich Beef Stock (here)

Direction:

- Preheat the oven to 325°F. Season the beef ribs on all sides with salt and pepper.
- Place a deep ovenproof skillet over medium-high heat and add the olive oil.
- Sear the ribs on all sides until browned, about 6 minutes in total.
- Transfer the ribs to a plate. Add the garlic to the skillet and sauté until translucent, about 3 minutes.
- Whisk in the red wine to deglaze the pan.
- Be sure to scrape all the browned bits from the meat from the

bottom of the pan.

- Simmer the wine until it is slightly reduced, about 2 minutes.
- Add the beef stock, ribs, and any accumulated juices on the plate back to the skillet and bring the liquid to a boil.
- Cover the skillet and place it in the oven to braise the ribs until the meat is fall-off-the-bone tender, about 2 hours.
- Serve the ribs with a spoonful of the cooking liquid drizzled over each serving.

Nutrition: Calories: 481 Fat: 38g Protein: 29g Carbs: 5g Fiber: 3g Net Carbs: 2g Fat 70%/Protein 25%/Carbs 5%

Pulled Pork

Servings: 8 Cooking Time: 2½ Hours

Ingredients:

- 2 tablespoons chili powder
- teaspoon garlic powder
- ½ teaspoon onion powder
- ½ teaspoon ground black pepper
- ½ teaspoon cumin

Direction:

- (4-pound) pork shoulder In a small bowl, mix chili powder, garlic powder, onion powder, pepper, and cumin.
- Rub the spice mixture over the pork shoulder, patting it into the skin.
- Place pork shoulder into the air fryer basket.
- Adjust the temperature to 350°F and set the timer for 150 minutes.
- Pork skin will be crispy and meat easily shredded with two forks when done.
- The internal temperature should be at least 145°F.

Nutrition: Calories: 537 Protein: 42.6 G Fiber: 0.8 G Net Carbohydrates: 0.7 G Fat: 35.5 G Sodium: 180 Mg Carbohydrates: 1.5 G Sugar: 0.2 G

Rosemary-garlic Lamb Racks

Servings: 4 Cooking Time: 25 Minutes

Ingredients:

- 4 tablespoons extra-virgin olive oil
- 2 tablespoons finely chopped fresh rosemary
- 2 teaspoons minced garlic Pinch sea salt
- 2 (1-pound) racks
- French-cut lamb chops (8 bones each)

Direction:

- In a small bowl, whisk together the olive oil, rosemary, garlic, and salt. Place the racks in a sealable freezer bag and pour the olive oil mixture into the bag.
- Massage the meat through the bag so it is coated with the marinade. Press the air out of the bag and seal it. Marinate the lamb racks in the refrigerator for 1 to 2 hours. Preheat the oven to 450°F. Place a large ovenproof skillet over medium-high heat.
- Take the lamb racks out of the bag and sear them in the skillet on all sides, about 5 minutes in total.
- Arrange the racks upright in the skillet, with the bones interlaced, and roast them in the oven until they reach your desired doneness, about 20 minutes for medium-rare or until

the internal temperature reaches 125°F.

- Let the lamb rest for 10 minutes and then cut the racks into chops. Serve 4 chops per person.

Nutrition: Calories: 354 Fat: 30g Protein: 21g Carbs: 0g Fiber: 0g Net Carbs: 0g Fat 70%/Protein 30%/Carbs 0%

Irish Pork Roast

Preparation Time: 40 minutes Cooking Time: 1 hour
Servings: 8

Ingredients:

- ½ lb. parsnips, peeled and sliced into small pieces
- ½ lb. carrots, sliced into small pieces
- 3 tablespoons olive oil, divided
- 2 teaspoons fresh thyme leaves, divided
- Salt and pepper to taste
- 2 lb. pork loin roast
- teaspoon honey
- cup dry hard cider Applesauce

Direction:

- Preheat your oven to 400 degrees F.
- Drizzle half of the oil over the parsnips and carrots. Season with half of thyme, salt and pepper.
- Arrange on a roasting pan. Rub the pork with the remaining oil.
- Season with the remaining thyme.
- Season with salt and pepper. Put it on the roasting pan on top of the vegetables.

- Roast for 65 minutes.
- Let cool before slicing.
- Transfer the carrots and parsnips in a bowl and mix with honey.
- Add the cider. Place in a pan and simmer over low heat until the sauce has thickened.
- Serve the pork with the vegetables and applesauce.

Nutrition: Calories 272 Total Fat 8 g Saturated Fat 2 g Cholesterol 61 mg Sodium 327 mg Total Carbohydrate 23 g Dietary Fiber 6 g Total Sugars 10 g Protein 24 g

Fish And Seafood

Herbed Salmon

Preparation Time: 10 minutes Cooking Time: 3 Minutes Servings: 4

Ingredients:

- 4 (4-ounce) salmon fillets
- ¼ cup olive oil
- 2 tablespoons fresh lemon juice
- 1 garlic clove, minced
- ¼ teaspoon dried oregano
- Salt and ground black pepper, as required
- 4 fresh rosemary sprigs
- 4 lemon slices

Direction:

- For dressing: in a large bowl, add oil, lemon juice, garlic, oregano, salt and black pepper and beat until well co combined.
- Arrange a steamer trivet in the Instant Pot and pour 11/2 cups of water in Instant Pot.
- Place the salmon fillets on top of trivet in a single layer and

top with dressing.

- Arrange 1 rosemary sprig and 1 lemon slice over each fillet. Close the lid and place the pressure valve to "Seal" position.
- Press "Steam" and just use the default time of 3 minutes.
- Press "Cancel" and carefully allow a "Quick" release.
- Open the lid and serve hot.

Nutrition: Calories 262, Fats 17g, Carbs 0.7g, Sugar 0.2g, Proteins 22.1g, Sodium 91mg

Salmon in Green Sauce

Preparation Time: 10 minutes Cooking Time: 12 Minutes Servings: 4

Ingredients:

- 4 (6-ounce) salmon fillets
- avocado, peeled, pitted and chopped
- 1/2 cup fresh basil, chopped
- 3 garlic cloves, chopped
- tablespoon fresh lemon zest, grated finely

Direction:

- Grease a large piece of foil.
- In a large bowl, add all ingredients except salmon and water and with a fork, mash completely.
- Place fillets in the center of foil and top with avocado mixture evenly.
- Fold the foil around fillets to seal them.
- Arrange a steamer trivet in the Instant Pot and pour 1/2 cup of water.
- Place the foil packet on top of trivet.
- Close the lid and place the pressure valve to "Seal" position.
- Press "Manual" and cook under "High Pressure" for about

minutes.

- Meanwhile, preheat the oven to broiler.
- Press "Cancel" and allow a "Natural" release.
- Open the lid and transfer the salmon fillets onto a broiler pan.
- Broil for about 3-4 minutes.
- Serve warm.

Nutrition: Calories 333, Fats 20.3g, Carbs 5.5g, Sugar 0.4g, Proteins 34.2g, Sodium 79mg

Braised Shrimp

Preparation Time: 10 minutes Cooking Time: 4 Minutes Servings: 4

Ingredients:

- pound frozen large shrimp, peeled and deveined
- 2 shallots, chopped
- ¾ cup low-sodium chicken broth
- 2 tablespoons fresh lemon juice
- 2 tablespoons olive oil
- tablespoon garlic, crushed
- Ground black pepper, as required

Direction:

- In the Instant Pot, place oil and press "Sauté". Now add the shallots and cook for about 2 minutes.
- Add the garlic and cook for about 1 minute.
- Press "Cancel" and stir in the shrimp, broth, lemon juice and black pepper.
- Close the lid and place the pressure valve to "Seal" position.
- Press "Manual" and cook under "High Pressure" for about 1 minute.

- Press "Cancel" and carefully allow a "Quick" release.
- Open the lid and serve hot.

Nutrition: Calories 209, Fats 9g, Carbs 4.3g, Sugar 0.2g, Proteins 26.6g, Sodium 293mg

Shrimp Coconut Curry

Preparation Time: 10 minutes Cooking Time: 20 Minutes Servings: 2

Ingredients:

- 0.5lb cooked shrimp
- thinly sliced onion
- 1 cup coconut yogurt
- 3tbsp curry paste
- 1tbsp oil or ghee

Direction:

- Set the Instant Pot to sauté and add the onion, oil, and curry paste.
- When the onion is soft, add the remaining ingredients and seal.
- Cook on Stew for 20 minutes.
- Release the pressure naturally.

Nutrition: Calories: 380 Carbs 13; Sugar 4; Fat 22; Protein 40; GL 14

DESSERTS

Raspberry Cake With White Chocolate Sauce

Preparation time: 15 minutes , Cooking time: 60 minutes Yield: 5-6 Servings

Ingredients:

- 5 Ounces of melted cacao butter
- 2 Ounces of grass-fed ghee
- 1/2 Cup of coconut cream
- Cup of green banana flour
- 3 Teaspoons of pure vanilla
- 4 Large eggs
- 1/2 Cup of as Lakanto Monk Fruit
- 1 Teaspoon of baking powder
- 2 Teaspoons of apple cider vinegar
- 2 Cup of raspberries
- For the white chocolate sauce:
- 3 and 1/2 ounces of cacao butter
- 1/2 Cup of coconut cream
- 2 Teaspoons of pure vanilla extract
- Pinch of salt

Direction:

- Preheat your oven to a temperature of about 280 degrees Fahrenheit.
- Combine the green banana flour with the pure vanilla extract, the baking powder, the coconut cream, the eggs, the cider vinegar and the monk fruit and mix very well.
- Leave the raspberries aside and line a cake loaf tin with a baking paper .
- Pour in the batter into the baking tray and scatter the raspberries over the top of the cake.
- Place the tray in your oven and bake it for about 60 minutes; in the meantime, prepare the sauce by Directions for sauce:
- Combine the cacao cream, the vanilla extract, the cacao butter and the salt in a saucepan over a low heat.
- Mix all your ingredients with a fork to make sure the cacao butter mixes very well with the cream.
- Remove from the heat and set aside to cool a little bit; but don't let it harden.
- Drizzle with the chocolate sauce.
- Scatter the cake with more raspberries.
- Slice your cake; then serve and enjoy it!

Nutrition: Calories: 323| Fat: 31.5g | Carbohydrates: 9.9g | Fiber: 4g |Protein: 5g

Ketogenic Lava Cake

Preparation time: 10 minutes, Cooking time: 10 minutes Yield: 2 Servings

Ingredients:

- 2 Oz of dark chocolate; you should at least use chocolate of 85% cocoa solids
- 1 Tablespoon of super-fine almond flour
- 2 Oz of unsalted almond butter
- 2 Large eggs

Direction:

- Heat your oven to a temperature of about 350 Fahrenheit.
- Grease 2 heat proof ramekins with almond butter.
- Now, melt the chocolate and the almond butter and stir very well.
- Beat the eggs very well with a mixer.
- Add the eggs to the chocolate and the butter mixture and mix very well with almond flour and the swerve; then stir.
- Pour the dough into 2 ramekins.
- Bake for about 9 to 10 minutes.
- Turn the cakes over plates and serve with pomegranate seeds!

Nutrition: Calories: 459| Fat: 39g | Carbohydrates: 3.5g | Fiber: 0.8g |Protein: 11.7g

Ketogenic Cheese Cake

Preparation time: 15 minutes, Cooking time: 50 minutes Yield: 6 Servings

Ingredients:

- For the Almond Flour Cheesecake Crust:
- 2 Cups of Blanched almond flour
- 1/3 Cup of almond Butter
- 3 Tablespoons of Erythritol (powdered or granular)
- 1 Teaspoon of Vanilla extract
- For the Keto Cheesecake Filling:
- 32 Oz of softened Cream cheese
- and ¼ cups of powdered erythritol
- 3 Large Eggs
- Tablespoon of Lemon juice
- Teaspoon of Vanilla extract

Direction:

- Preheat your oven to a temperature of about 350 degrees F.
- Grease a spring form pan of 9" with cooking spray or just line its bottom with a parchment paper.
- In order to make the cheesecake rust, stir in the melted butter, the almond flour, the vanilla extract and the erythritol in a large bowl.

- The dough will get will be a bit crumbly; so press it into the bottom of your prepared tray.
- Bake for about 12 minutes; then let cool for about 10 minutes.
- In the meantime, beat the softened cream cheese and the powdered sweetener at a low speed until it becomes smooth.
- Crack in the eggs and beat them in at a low to medium speed until it becomes fluffy. Make sure to add one a time.
- Add in the lemon juice and the vanilla extract and mix at a low to medium speed with a mixer.
- Pour your filling into your pan right on top of the crust. You can use a spatula to smooth the top of the cake.
- Bake for about 45 to 50 minutes.
- Remove the baked cheesecake from your oven and run a knife around its edge.
- Let the cake cool for about 4 hours in the refrigerator.
- Serve and enjoy your delicious cheese cake!

Nutrition: Calories: 325| Fat: 29g | Carbohydrates: 6g | Fiber: 1g |Protein: 7g

Cake with Whipped Cream Icing

Preparation time: 20 minutes, Cooking time: 25 minutes Yield: 7 Servings

Ingredients:

- ¾ Cup Coconut flour
- ¾ Cup of Swerve Sweetener
- 1/2 Cup of Cocoa powder
- 2 Teaspoons of Baking powder
- 6 Large Eggs
- 2/3 Cup of Heavy Whipping Cream
- 1/2 Cup of Melted almond Butter
- For the whipped Cream Icing:
- Cup of Heavy Whipping Cream
- ¼ Cup of Swerve Sweetener
- Teaspoon of Vanilla extract
- 1/3 Cup of Sifted Cocoa Powder

Direction:

- Pre-heat your oven to a temperature of about 350 F.
- Grease an 8x8 cake tray with cooking spray.
- Add the coconut flour, the Swerve sweetener; the cocoa powder, the baking powder, the eggs, the melted butter; and combine very well with an electric or a hand mixer.

- Pour your batter into the cake tray and bake for about 25 minutes.
- Remove the cake tray from the oven and let cool for about 5 minutes.

✓ For the Icing:

- Whip the cream until it becomes fluffy; then add in the Swerve, the vanilla and the cocoa powder.
- Add the Swerve, the vanilla and the cocoa powder; then continue mixing until your ingredients are very well combined.
- Frost your baked cake with the icing; then slice it; serve and enjoy your delicious cake!

Nutrition: Calories: 357| Fat: 33g | Carbohydrates: 11g | Fiber: 2g |Protein: 8g

Walnut-Fruit Cake

Ingredients:

- 1/2 Cup of almond butter (softened)
- ¼ Cup of so Nourished granulated erythritol
- Tablespoon of ground cinnamon
- 1/2 Teaspoon of ground nutmeg
- ¼ Teaspoon of ground cloves
- 4 Large pastured eggs
- 1 Teaspoon of vanilla extract
- 1/2 Teaspoon of almond extract
- 2 Cups of almond flour
- 1/2 Cup of chopped walnuts
- ¼ Cup of dried of unsweetened cranberries
- ¼ Cup of seedless raisins

Direction:

- Preheat your oven to a temperature of about 350 F and grease an 8-inch baking tin of round shape with coconut oil.
- Beat the granulated erythritol on a high speed until it becomes fluffy.
- Add the cinnamon, the nutmeg, and the cloves; then blend your ingredients until they become smooth.

- Crack in the eggs and beat very well by adding one at a time, plus the almond extract and the vanilla.
- Whisk in the almond flour until it forms a smooth batter then fold in the nuts and the fruit.
- Spread your mixture into your prepared baking pan and bake it for about 20 minutes.
- Remove the cake from the oven and let cool for about 5 minutes.
- Dust the cake with the powdered erythritol.
- Serve and enjoy your cake!

Nutrition: Calories: 250| Fat: 11g | Carbohydrates: 12g | Fiber: 2g |Protein: 7g

More Recipes

Tabbouleh- Arabian Salad

Preparation time: 5 minutes Cooking time: 10 minutes Servings: 6

Ingredients:

- ¼ cup chopped fresh mint
- 2/3 cups boiling water
- cucumber, peeled, seeded and chopped
- cup bulgur
- 1 cup chopped fresh parsley
- 1 cup chopped green onions
- tsp. salt
- 1/3 cup lemon juice
- 1/3 cup olive oil
- 3 tomatoes, chopped
- Ground black pepper to taste

Direction:

- In a large bowl, mix together boiling water and bulgur. Let soak and set aside for an hour while covered.
- After one hour, toss in cucumber, tomatoes, mint, parsley,

onions, lemon juice and oil. Then season with black pepper and salt to taste. Toss well and refrigerate for another hour while covered before serving.

Nutrition: Calories: 185.5g fat: 13.1g Protein: 4.1g Carbs: 12.8g

Cheese Stuff Peppers

Time: 13 minutes - Serve: 8

Ingredients:

- 8 small bell pepper, cut the top of peppers
- 3.5 oz feta cheese, cubed
- 1 tbsp olive oil 1 tsp Italian seasoning
- 1 tbsp parsley, chopped
- ¼ tsp garlic powder
- Pepper Salt

Direction:

- In a bowl, toss cheese with oil and seasoning.
- Stuff cheese in each bell peppers and place into the air fryer basket.
- Cook at 400 F for 8 minutes.
- Serve and enjoy.

Roasted Pepper Salad

Time: 20 minutes - Serve: 4

Ingredients:

- 4 bell peppers
- 2 oz rocket leaves
- 2 tbsp olive oil
- 4 tbsp heavy cream
- lettuce head, torn
- tbsp fresh lime juice
- Pepper Salt

Direction:

- Add bell peppers into the air fryer basket and cook for 10 minutes at 400 F.
- Remove peppers from air fryer and let it cool for 5 minutes.
- Peel cooked peppers and cut into strips and place into the large bowl.
- Add remaining ingredients into the bowl and toss well.
- Serve.

Breakfast Casserole Delicious

Time: 30 minutes - Serve: 4

Ingredients:

- 4 eggs
- 7 oz spinach, chopped
- 3 bacon slices, chopped
- 8 grape tomatoes, halved
- 1 garlic clove, minced
- 8 mushrooms, sliced
- Pepper Salt

Direction:

- Spray air fryer baking dish with cooking spray and set aside.
- Add all ingredients into the large bowl and whisk until well combined.
- Pour bowl mixture into the prepared baking dish.
- Place dish in the air fryer and cook at 400 F for 20 minutes.
- Serve.

Huevos Rancheros

Ingredients:

- 4 large eggs
- ¼ teaspoon kosher salt
- ¼ cup masa harina (corn flour)
- 1 teaspoon olive oil
- ¼ cup warm water
- ½ cup salsa
- ¼ cup crumbled queso fresco or feta cheese

Direction: Time: 45 minutes | Serves 4

- Crack the eggs into a baking pan, season with the kosher salt, and bake at 330°F (166°C) for 3 minutes.
- Pause the fryer, gently scramble the eggs, and bake for 2 more minutes.
- Remove the eggs from the fryer, keeping the fryer on, and set the eggs aside to slightly cool. (Clean the baking pan before making the tortillas.)
- Increase the temperature to 390°F (199°C).
- In a medium bowl, combine the masa harina, olive oil, and ¼ teaspoon of kosher salt by hand, then slowly pour in the water, stirring until a soft dough forms.

- Divide the dough into 4 equal balls, then place each ball between 2 pieces of parchment paper and use a pie plate or a rolling pin to flatten the dough.
- Spray the baking pan with nonstick cooking spray, then place one flattened tortilla in the pan and air fry for 5 minutes.
- Repeat this process with the remaining tortillas.
- Remove the tortillas from the fryer and place on a serving plate, then top each tortilla with the scrambled eggs, salsa, and cheese before serving.
- Yummy

Flourless Broccoli Cheese Quiche

Time: 55 minutes | Servings: 2

Ingredients:

- large broccoli
- 3 large carrots
- tsp thyme
- tsp parsley
- Salt and ground black pepper to taste
- 2 large eggs
- 5 oz whole milk
- large tomato
- 4 oz cheddar cheese grated
- oz feta cheese

Direction:

- Chop up your broccoli into florets.
- Then dice your peeled carrots and combine it with the broccoli in a food steamer.
- Allow cooking until soft (for about 20 minutes).
- Get a measuring cup, and in it, combine all the seasonings, and crack the eggs into it as well.
- Mix thoroughly before adding the milk gradually until the mixture is pale.

- After steaming, drain the vegetables and use it to line the base of your quiche dish.
- Layer with the tomatoes and then add your cheese on top.
- Pour the liquid over and then add a little bit more cheese on top.
- Transfer the liquid into the fryer and allow to cook for 20 minutes at 360 F.
- Serve.

Asparagus Cheese Strata

Time: 30 minutes | Serves 4-6

Ingredients:

- asparagus spears, cut into 2-inch pieces
- 2 slices whole-wheat bread, cut into ½-inch cubes
- 4 eggs
- 3 tbls whole milk
- ½ cup grated Havarti or Swiss cheese
- 2 tablespoons chopped flat-leaf parsley
- Pinch salt
- Freshly ground black pepper, to taste

Direction:

- Place the asparagus spears and 1 tablespoon water in a baking pan and place in the air fryer basket.
- Bake at 330°F (166°C) for 3 to 5 minutes or until crisp and tender.
- Remove the asparagus from the pan and drain it.
- Spray the pan with nonstick cooking spray.
- Arrange the bread cubes and asparagus into the pan and set aside.
- In a medium bowl, beat the eggs with the milk until combined.

- Add the cheese, parsley, salt, and pepper.
- Pour into the baking pan. Bake for 11 to 14 minutes or until the eggs are set and the top starts to brown.
- Serve

Almond Crunch Granola

Time: 8 to 10 minutes | Makes 1

Ingredients:

- ⅓ cups
- ⅔ cup rolled oats
- ⅓ cup unsweetened shredded coconut
- ⅓ cup sliced almonds
- teaspoon canola oil
- 2 teaspoons honey
- ¼ teaspoon kosher salt

Direction:

- In a medium bowl, combine the rolled oats, shredded coconut, sliced almonds, canola oil, honey, and kosher salt.
- Place a small piece of parchment paper on the bottom of a baking pan, then pour the mixture into the pan and distribute it evenly.
- Bake at 360°F (182°C) for 5 minutes, pause the fryer to gently stir the granola, and bake for 3 more minutes.
- Remove the granola from the fryer and allow to cool in the pan on a wire rack for 5 minutes, then transfer the granola to a serving plate to cool completely before serving.
- Enjoy

✓ Tips:

- (It becomes crunchier as it cools. Store the granola in an airtight container for up to 2 weeks.)

Vegetable Frittata

Prep time: 25-30 minutes | Serves 4

Ingredients:

- ½ cup chopped red bell pepper
- ⅓ cup minced onion
- ⅓ cup grated carrot
- 1 teaspoon olive oil
- 6 egg whites
- egg
- ⅓ cup 2% milk
- tablespoon grated Parmesan cheese

Direction:

- In a baking pan, stir together the red bell pepper, onion, carrot, and olive oil.
- Put the pan into the air fryer.
- Bake at 350°F (177°C) for 4 to 6 minutes, shaking the basket once, until the vegetables are tender.
- Meanwhile, in a medium bowl, beat the egg whites, egg, and milk until combined.
- Pour the egg mixture over the vegetables in the pan.
- Sprinkle with the Parmesan cheese.
- Return the pan to the air fryer.

- Bake for 4 to 6 minutes more, or until the frittata is puffy and set.
- Cut into 4 wedges
- serve.

Breakfast Burrito

Time: 13 to 15 minutes | Serves 4

Ingredients:

- 2 hard-boiled egg whites, chopped
- hard-boiled egg, chopped
- 1 avocado, peeled, pitted, and chopped
- 1 red bell pepper, chopped
- 3 tablespoons low-sodium salsa,
- additional for serving(optional):
- (1.2-ounce / 34-g) slice low-sodium, low-fat American cheese, torn into pieces
- 4 low-sodium whole-wheat flour tortillas

Direction:

- In a medium bowl, thoroughly mix the egg whites, egg, avocado, red bell pepper, salsa, and cheese.
- Place the tortillas on a work surface and evenly divide the filling among them.
- Fold in the edges and roll up.
- Secure the burritos with toothpicks if necessary.
- Put the burritos in the air fryer basket.
- Air fry at 390°F (199°C) for 3 to 5 minutes, or until the burritos are light golden brown and crisp.

- Serve with more salsa if desired

Pumpkin Oatmeal with Raisins

Time: 10 minutes | Makes 3 cups

Ingredients:

- cup rolled oats
- 2 tablespoons raisins
- ¼ teaspoon ground cinnamon
- Pinch of kosher salt
- ¼ cup pumpkin purée
- 2 tablespoons pure maple syrup
- cup low-fat milk

Direction:

- In a medium bowl, combine the rolled oats, raisins, ground cinnamon, and kosher salt, then stir in the pumpkin purée, maple syrup, and low-fat milk.
- Spray a baking pan with nonstick cooking spray, then pour the oatmeal mixture into the pan and bake at 300°F (149°C) for 10 minutes.
- Remove the oatmeal from the fryer and allow to cool in the pan on a wire rack for 5 minutes
- Serve

Mushroom and Black Bean Burrito

Time: 15 minutes | Serves 1

Ingredients:

- 2 tablespoons canned black beans, rinsed and drained
- ¼ cup sliced baby portobello mushrooms
- teaspoon olive oil
- Pinch of kosher salt
- 1 large egg
- slice low-fat Cheddar cheese
- (8-inch) whole grain flour tortilla
- Hot sauce (optional)

Direction:

- Spray a baking pan with nonstick cooking spray, then place the black beans and baby portobello mushrooms in the pan, drizzle with the olive oil, and season with the kosher salt.
- Bake at 360°F (182°C) for 5 minutes, then pause the fryer to crack the egg on top of the beans and mushrooms.
- Bake for 8 more minutes or until the egg is cooked as desired.
- Pause the fryer again, top the egg with cheese, and bake for 1 more minute.
- Remove the pan from the fryer, then use a spatula to place

the bean mixture on the whole grain flour tortilla.
- Fold in the sides and roll from front to back.
- Serve warm with the hot sauce on the side (if using).

Shrimp with Green Beans

Preparation Time: 10 minutes Cooking Time: 2 Minutes Servings: 4

Ingredients:

- ¾ pound fresh green beans, trimmed
- pound medium frozen shrimp, peeled and deveined
- 2 tablespoons fresh lemon juice
- 2 tablespoons olive oil
- Salt and ground black pepper, as required

Direction:

- Arrange a steamer trivet in the Instant Pot and pour cup of water.
- Arrange the green beans on top of trivet in a single layer and top with shrimp.
- Drizzle with oil and lemon juice.
- Sprinkle with salt and black pepper.
- Close the lid and place the pressure valve to "Seal" position.
- Press "Steam" and just use the default time of 2 minutes.
- Press "Cancel" and allow a "Natural" release.
- Open the lid and serve.

Nutrition: Calories 223, Fats 1g, Carbs 7.9g, Sugar 1.4g, Proteins 27.4g, Sodium 322mg

Crab Curry

Preparation Time: 10 minutes Cooking Time: 20 Minutes Servings: 2

Ingredients:

- 0.5lb chopped crab
- thinly sliced red onion
- 0.5 cup chopped tomato 3tbsp curry paste
- 1tbsp oil or ghee

Direction:

- Set the Instant Pot to sauté and add the onion, oil, and curry paste.
- When the onion is soft, add the remaining ingredients and seal.
- Cook on Stew for 20 minutes.
- Release the pressure naturally.

Nutrition: Calories 2; Carbs 11; Sugar 4; Fat 10; Protein 24; GL 9

Mixed Chowder

Preparation Time: 10 minutes Cooking Time: 35 Minutes Servings: 2

Ingredients:

- 1lb fish stew mix
- 2 cups white sauce
- 3tbsp old bay seasoning

Direction:

- Mix all the ingredients in your Instant Pot.
- Cook on Stew for 35 minutes.
- Release the pressure naturally.

Nutrition:: Calories 320; Carbs 9; Sugar 2; Fat 16; Protein GL 4

Mussels in Tomato Sauce

Preparation Time: 10 minutes Cooking Time: 3 Minutes Servings: 4

Ingredients:

- 2 tomatoes, seeded and chopped finely
- 2 pounds mussels, scrubbed and de-bearded
- 1 cup low-sodium chicken broth
- 1 tablespoon fresh lemon juice
- 2 garlic cloves, minced

Direction:

- In the pot of Instant Pot, place tomatoes, garlic, wine and bay leaf and stir to combine.
- Arrange the mussels on top.
- Close the lid and place the pressure valve to "Seal" position.
- Press "Manual" and cook under "High Pressure" for about 3 minutes.
- Press "Cancel" and carefully allow a "Quick" release.
- Open the lid and serve hot.

Nutrition: Calories 213, Fats 25.2g, Carbs 11g, Sugar 1. Proteins 28.2g, Sodium 670mg

Citrus Salmon

Preparation Time: 10 minutes Cooking Time: 7 Minutes Servings: 4

Ingredients:

- 4 (4-ounce) salmon fillets
- cup low-sodium chicken broth
- teaspoon fresh ginger, minced
- 2 teaspoons fresh orange zest, grated finely
- 3 tablespoons fresh orange juice
- tablespoon olive oil
- Ground black pepper, as required

Direction:

- In Instant Pot, add all ingredients and mix.
- Close the lid and place the pressure valve to "Seal" position.
- Press "Manual" and cook under "High Pressure" for about 7 minutes.
- Press "Cancel" and allow a "Natural" release.
- Open the lid and serve the salmon fillets with the topping of cooking sauce.

Nutrition: Calories 190, Fats 10.5g, Carbs 1.8g, Sugar 1g, Proteins 22. Sodium 68mg

Pork with Bell Peppers

Preparation Time: 15 minutes Cooking Time: 13 minutes Servings: 4

Ingredients:

- tablespoon fresh ginger, chopped finely
- 4 garlic cloves, chopped finely
- cup fresh cilantro, chopped and divided
- ¼ cup plus
- 1 tablespoon olive oil, divided
- 1 pound tender pork, trimmed, sliced thinly
- 2 onions, sliced thinly
- green bell pepper, seeded and sliced thinly
- red bell pepper, seeded and sliced thinly
- tablespoon fresh lime juice

Direction:

- In a large bowl, mix together ginger, garlic, ½ cup of cilantro and ¼ cup of oil.
- Add the pork and coat with mixture generously.
- Refrigerate to marinate for about 2 hours.
- Heat a large skillet over medium-high heat and stir fry the pork mixture for about 4-5 minutes.

- Transfer the pork into a bowl. In the same skillet, heat remaining oil over medium heat and sauté the onion for about 3 minutes. Stir in the bell pepper and stir fry for about 3 minutes.
- Stir in the pork, lime juice and remaining cilantro and cook for about 2 minutes.
- Serve hot.
- Meal Prep Tip:
- Transfer the pork mixture into a large bowl and set aside to cool.
- Divide the mixture into 4 containers evenly.
- Cover the containers and refrigerate for 1-2 days. Reheat in the microwave before serving

Nutrition: Calories 360 Total Fat 21.8 g Saturated Fat 3.9 g Cholesterol 83 mg Total Carbs 11 g Sugar 5.4 g Fiber 2.2 g Sodium 71 mg Potassium 706 mg Protein 31.2 g

Roasted Pork Shoulder

Preparation Time: 10 minutes **Cooking Time:** 6 hours
Servings: 12

Ingredients:

- head garlic, peeled and crushed
- ¼ cup fresh rosemary, minced
- 2 tablespoons fresh lemon juice
- 2 tablespoons balsamic vinegar
- (4-pound) pork shoulder, trimmed

Direction:

- In a bowl, add all the ingredients except pork shoulder and mix well.
- In a large roasting pan place pork shoulder and coat with marinade generously.
- With a large plastic wrap, cover the roasting pan and refrigerate to marinate for at least 1-2 hours.
- Remove the roasting pan from refrigerator.
- Remove the plastic wrap from roasting pan and keep in room temperature for 1 hour. Preheat the oven to 275 degrees F. Arrange the roasting pan in oven and roast for about 6 hours.
- Remove from the oven and set aside for about 15-20 minutes.

With a sharp knife, cut the pork shoulder into desired slices and serve.

- Meal Prep Tip:
- Transfer the pork slices onto a wire rack to cool completely. With foil pieces, wrap the pork slices and refrigerate for about 1-2 days. Reheat in the microwave before serving.

Nutrition: Calories 450 Total Fat 32.6g Saturated Fat 12 g Cholesterol 136 mg Total Carbs 1.5 g Sugar 0.1 g Fiber 0.6 g Sodium 104 mg Potassium 522 mg Protein 35.4 g

Pork Chops in Peach Glaze

Preparation Time: 15 minutes Cooking Time: 16 minutes Servings: 2

Ingredients:

- 2 (6-ounce) boneless pork chops, trimmed
- Sea Salt and ground black pepper, as required
- ½ of ripe yellow peach, peeled, pitted and chopped
- 1 tablespoon olive oil
- 2 tablespoons shallot, minced
- 2 tablespoons garlic, minced
- 2 tablespoons fresh ginger, minced
- 4-6 drops liquid stevia
- tablespoon balsamic vinegar
- ¼ teaspoon red pepper flakes, crushed
- ¼ cup filtered water

Direction:

- Season the pork chops with sea salt and black pepper generously.
- In a blender, add the peach pieces and pulse until a puree forms.
- Reserve the remaining peach pieces. In a skillet, heat the oil

over medium heat and sauté the shallots for about 1-2 minutes.

- Add the garlic and ginger and sauté for about 1 minute. Stir in the remaining ingredients and bring to a boil.
- Now, reduce the heat to medium-low and simmer for about 4-5 minutes or until a sticky glaze forms.
- Remove from the heat and reserve 1/3 of the glaze and set aside. Coat the chops with remaining glaze.
- Heat a nonstick skillet over medium-high heat and sear the chops for about 4 minutes per side.
- Transfer the chops onto a plate and coat with the remaining glaze evenly.
- Serve immediately.
- Meal Prep Tip:
- Transfer the pork chops into a large bowl and set aside to cool.
- Divide the chops into 2 containers evenly.
- Cover the containers and refrigerate for 1-2 days. Reheat in the microwave before serving.

Nutrition: Calories 359 Total Fat 13.5 g Saturated Fat 3.2 g Cholesterol 124 mg Total Carbs 12 g Sugar 3.8 g Fiber 1.5 g Sodium 102 mg Potassium 938 mg Protein 46.2 g

Ground Pork with Spinach

Preparation Time: 15 minutes **Cooking Time:** 15 minutes **Servings:** 4

Ingredients:

- tablespoon olive oil
- ½ of white onion, chopped
- 2 garlic cloves, chopped finely
- jalapeño pepper, chopped finely
- pound lean ground pork
- teaspoon ground coriander
- 1 teaspoon ground cumin
- ½ teaspoon ground turmeric
- ½ teaspoon ground cinnamon
- ½ teaspoon ground fennel seeds
- Salt and ground black pepper, as required
- ½ cup fresh cherry tomatoes, quartered
- 1¼ pounds collard greens leaves, stemmed and chopped
- teaspoon fresh lemon juice

Direction:

- In a large skillet, heat the oil over medium heat and sauté the onion for about 4 minutes.

- Add the garlic and jalapeño pepper and sauté for about 1 minute.
- Add the pork and spices and cook for about 6 minutes breaking into pieces with the spoon.
- Stir in the tomatoes and greens and cook, stirring gently for about 4 minutes. Stir in the lemon juice and remove from heat. Serve hot.
- Meal Prep Tip:
- Transfer the pork mixture into a large bowl and set aside to cool. Divide the mixture into 4 containers evenly. Cover the containers and refrigerate for 1-2 days. Reheat in the microwave before serving.

Nutrition: Calories 316 Total Fat 21.8 g Saturated Fat 0.5 g Cholesterol 0 mg Total Carbs 11.4 g Sugar 1.4 g Fiber 5.7 g Sodium 27 mg Potassium 107 mg Protein 23 g

Yogurt Raspberry Cake

Time: 18 minutes | Makes 4 slices

Ingredients:

- ½ cup whole wheat pastry flour
- ⅛ teaspoon kosher salt
- ¼ teaspoon baking powder
- ½ cup whole milk vanilla yogurt
- 2 tablespoons canola oil
- 2 tablespoons pure maple syrup
- ¾ cup fresh raspberries

Direction:

- In a large bowl, combine the whole wheat pastry flour, kosher salt, and baking powder, then stir in the whole milk vanilla yogurt, canola oil, and maple syrup and gently fold in the raspberries.
- Spray a baking pan with nonstick cooking spray, then pour the cake batter into the pan and bake at 300°F (149°C) for 8 minutes.
- Remove the cake from the fryer and allow to cool in the pan on a wire rack for 10 minutes before cutting and serving.

Turkey Egg Casserole

Time: 35 minutes - Serve: 6

Ingredients:

- 12 eggs
- 2 tomatoes, chopped
- cup spinach, chopped
- ½ sweet potato, cubed
- 1 tsp chili powder
- tbsp olive oil
- lb ground turkey
- Pepper Salt

Direction:

- In a bowl, whisk eggs with pepper, chili powder, and salt until well combined.
- Add spinach, sweet potato, tomato, and turkey and stir well.
- Pour egg mixture into the air fryer baking dish and place in the air fryer.
- Cook at 350 F for 25 minutes.
- Serve.

Mixed Berry Dutch Pancake

time: 26 to 28 minutes | Serves 4

Ingredients:

- 2 egg whites
- egg
- ½ cup whole-wheat pastry flour
- ½ cup 2% milk
- 1 teaspoon pure vanilla extract
- 1 tablespoon unsalted butter, melted
- cup sliced fresh strawberries
- ½ cup fresh blueberries
- ½ cup fresh raspberries

Direction:

- In a medium bowl, use an eggbeater or hand mixer to quickly mix the egg whites, egg, pastry flour, milk, and vanilla until well combined.
- Use a pastry brush to grease the bottom of a baking pan with the melted butter.
- Immediately pour in the batter and put the baking pan in the fryer.
- Bake at 330°F (166°C) for 12 to 16 minutes, or until the pancake is puffed and golden brown.

- Remove the pan from the air fryer; the pancake will fall.
- Top with the strawberries, blueberries, and raspberries.
- Serve immediately.

Jalapeño Potato Hash

Ingredients:

- 2 large sweet potatoes
- ½ small red onion, cut into large chunks
- green bell pepper, cut into large chunks
- 1 jalapeño pepper, seeded and sliced
- ½ teaspoon kosher salt
- ¼ teaspoon freshly ground black pepper,
- extra for serving:
- teaspoon olive oil
- large egg.

Direction: Time: 30 minutes | Makes 4 cups

- poached Cook the sweet potatoes on high in the microwave until softened but not completely cooked (3 to 4 minutes), then set aside to cool for 10 minutes.
- Remove the skins from the sweet potatoes, then cut the sweet potatoes into large chunks.
- In a large bowl, combine the sweet potatoes, red onion, green bell pepper, jalapeño pepper, kosher salt, black pepper, and olive oil, tossing gently.
- Spray the air fryer basket with nonstick cooking spray, then

pour the mixture into the basket and air fry at 360°F (182°C) for 8 minutes.

- Pause the fryer to shake the basket, then air fry for 8 more minutes or until golden brown.
- Remove the hash from the fryer, place on a plate lined with a paper towel, and allow to cool for 5 minutes, then add the poached egg, sprinkle black pepper on top.
- Serve

Bacon and Egg Sandwiches

Time: 10 minutes | Makes 2 sandwiches

Ingredients:

- 2 large eggs
- ¼ teaspoon kosher salt, divided
- ¼ teaspoon freshly ground black pepper, divided
- plus extra for serving:
- 2 slices Canadian bacon
- 2 slices American cheese
- 2 whole grain English muffins, sliced in half

Direction:

- Spray two 3-inch ramekins with nonstick cooking spray, then crack one egg into each ramekin and add half the kosher salt and half the black pepper to each egg.
- Place the ramekins in the fryer basket and bake at 360°F (182°C) for 5 minutes.
- Pause the fryer and top each partially cooked egg with a slice of Canadian bacon and a slice of American cheese. Bake for 3 more minutes or until the cheese has melted and the egg yolk has just cooked through.
- Remove the ramekins from the fryer and allow to cool on a wire rack for 2 to 3 minutes, then flip the eggs, bacon, and cheese out onto English muffins and sprinkle some black

pepper on top.

- Serve

Spinach and Tomato Egg Cup

Time: 10 minutes | Serves 1

Ingredients:

- 2 egg whites, beaten
- 2 tablespoons chopped tomato
- 2 tablespoons chopped spinach
- Pinch of kosher salt
- Red pepper flakes (optional)

Direction:

- Spray a 3-inch ramekin with nonstick cooking spray, then combine the egg whites, tomato, spinach, kosher salt, and red pepper flakes (if using) in the ramekin.
- Place the ramekin in the air fryer basket and bake at 300°F (149°C) for 10 minutes or until the eggs have set.
- Remove the ramekin from the fryer and allow to cool on a wire rack for 5 minutes before serving.

Egg Muffins with Bell Pepper

Time: 10 minutes | Serves 2

Ingredients:

- 4 large eggs
- ½ bell pepper, finely chopped
- 1 tablespoon finely chopped red onion
- ¼ teaspoon kosher salt
- ¼ teaspoon freshly ground black pepper,
- extra for serving:
- 2 tablespoons shredded Cheddar cheese

Direction:

- In a large bowl, whisk together the eggs, then stir in the bell pepper, red onion, kosher salt, and black pepper.
- Spray two 3-inch ramekins with nonstick cooking spray, then pour half the egg mixture into each ramekin and place the ramekins in the fryer basket.
- Bake at 390°F (199°C) for 8 minutes.
- Pause the fryer, sprinkle 1 tablespoon of shredded Cheddar cheese on top of each cup, and bake for 2 more minutes.
- Remove the ramekins from the fryer and allow to cool on a wire rack for 5 minutes, then turn the omelet cups out on

plates and sprinkle some black pepper on top
- serve

Tomato and Spinach Egg Cup

Time: 10 minutes | Serves 1

Ingredients:

- 2 egg whites, beaten
- 2 tablespoons chopped tomato
- 2 tablespoons chopped spinach
- Pinch of kosher salt
- Red pepper flakes (optional)

Direction:

- Spray a 3-inch ramekin with nonstick cooking spray, then combine the egg whites, tomato, spinach, kosher salt, and red pepper flakes (if using) in the ramekin. Place the ramekin in the air fryer basket and bake at 300°F (149°C) for 10 minutes or until the eggs have set.
- Remove the ramekin from the fryer and allow to cool on a wire rack for 5 minutes
- Serve

Egg and Cheese Pockets

Time: 35 minutes | Makes 4 pockets

Ingredients:

- large egg, beaten
- Pinch of kosher salt
- ½ sheet puff pastry
- slice Cheddar cheese, divided into 4 pieces

Direction:

- Pour the egg into a baking pan, season with the kosher salt, and bake at 330°F (166°C) for 3 minutes.
- Pause the fryer, gently scramble the egg, and bake for 2 more minutes.
- Remove the egg from the fryer, keeping the fryer on, and set the egg aside to slightly cool.
- Roll the puff pastry out flat and divide into 4 pieces. Place a piece of Cheddar cheese and ¼ of the egg on one side of a piece of pastry, fold the pastry over the egg and cheese, and use a fork to press the edges closed.
- Repeat this process with the remaining pieces.
- Place 2 pockets in the fryer and bake for 15 minutes or until golden brown.
- Repeat this process with the other 2 pockets.

- Remove the pockets from the fryer and allow to cool on a wire rack for 5 minutes
- Serve

Leftovers Bubble and Squeak

Cooking Time: 30 minutes | Servings: 4

Ingredients:

- leftover vegetables (mash veggie bake, sprouts, cabbage, stuffing)
- tbsp mixed herbs
- 1 tsp tarragon
- Salt and ground black pepper to taste
- 2 oz Cheddar cheese, shredded
- medium onion, peeled and sliced
- 2 medium eggs, beaten
- 4 slices turkey breast

Direction:

- Get a large mixing bowl, and in it, place the leftovers, breaking them into small bits to facilitate blending.
- To the mixture, add the seasoning, cheese, onions, and eggs.
- Chop up the turkey and add it to the bowl and mix thoroughly using the hands.
- Transfer the mixture into ramekins or a baking dish and then into the air fryer.
- Allow cooking for 25 minutes at 360 F.
- Remove when it is bubbling on top. Serve.

Conclusion

Thank you for making it to the end. The warning symptoms of diabetes type 1 are the same as type 2; however, in type 1, these signs and symptoms tend to occur slowly over a period of months or years, making it harder to spot and recognize. Some of these symptoms can even occur after the disease has progressed.

Each disorder has risk factors that when found in an individual, favor the development of the disease. Diabetes is no different. Here are some of the risk factors for developing diabetes.

Having a Family History of Diabetes

Usually having a family member, especially first-degree relatives could be an indicator that you are at risk of developing diabetes. Your risk of developing diabetes is about 15% if you have one parent with diabetes while it is 75% if both your parents have diabetes.

Having Prediabetes

Being pre-diabetic means that you have higher than normal blood glucose levels. However, they are not high enough to be diagnosed as type 2 diabetes. Having pre-diabetes is a risk factor for developing type 2 diabetes as well as other conditions such as cardiac conditions. Since there are no symptoms or signs for Prediabetes, it is often a latent condition that is discovered accidentally during routine investigations of blood glucose levels or when investigating other conditions.

Being Obese or Overweight

Your metabolism, fat stores and eating habits when you are overweight or above the healthy weight range contribute to abnormal metabolism pathways that put you at risk for developing diabetes type 2. There have been consistent research results of the obvious link between developing diabetes and being obese.

Having a Sedentary Lifestyle

Having a lifestyle where you are mostly physically inactive predisposes you to a lot of conditions including diabetes type 2. That is because being physically inactive causes you to develop obesity or become overweight. Moreover, you don't burn any excess sugars that you ingest which can lead you to become prediabetic and eventually diabetic.

Having Gestational Diabetes

Developing gestational diabetes which is diabetes that occurred due to pregnancy (and often disappears after pregnancy) is a risk factor for developing diabetes at some point.

Ethnicity

Belonging to certain ethnic groups such as Middle Eastern, South Asian or Indian background. Studies of statistics have revealed that the prevalence of diabetes type 2 in these ethnic groups is high. If you come from any of these ethnicities, this puts you at risk of developing diabetes type 2 yourself.

Having Hypertension

Studies have shown an association between having hypertension and having an increased risk of developing diabetes. If you have hypertension, you should not leave it uncontrolled.

Extremes of Age

Diabetes can occur at any age. However, being too young or too old means your body is not in its best form and therefore, this increases the risk of developing diabetes.

That sounds scary. However, diabetes only occurs with the presence of a combination of these risk factors. Most of the risk factors can be minimized by taking action. For example, developing a more active lifestyle, taking care of your habits and attempting to lower your blood glucose sugar by restricting your sugar intake. If you start to notice you are prediabetic or getting overweight, etc., there is always something you can do to modify the situation. Recent studies show that developing healthy eating habits and following diets that are low in carbs, losing excess weight and leading an active lifestyle can help to protect you from developing diabetes, especially diabetes type 2, by minimizing the risk factors of developing the disorder.

You can also have an oral glucose tolerance test in which you will have a fasting glucose test first and then you will be given a sugary drink and then having your blood glucose tested 2 hours after that to see how your body responds to glucose meals. In healthy individuals, blood glucose should drop again 2 hours post sugary meals due to the action of insulin.

Another indicative test is the HbA1C. This test reflects the average of your blood glucose level over the last 2 to 3 months. It is also a test to see how well you manage your diabetes.

People with diabetes type 1 require compulsory insulin shots to control their diabetes because they have no other option. People with diabetes type 2 can regulate their diabetes with healthy eating and regular physical activity although they may require some glucose-lowering medications that can be in tablet form or in the form of an injection.

All the above goes in the direction that you need to avoid a starchy diet because of its tendency to raise blood glucose levels. Too many carbohydrates can lead to insulin sensitivity and pancreatic fatigue, as well as weight gain with all its associated risk factors for cardiovascular disease and hypertension. The solution is to lower your sugar intake, therefore, decrease your body's need for insulin and increase the burning of fat in your body.

When your body is low on sugars, it will be forced to use a subsequent molecule to burn for energy, in that case, this will be fat. The burning of fat will lead you to lose weight.

I hope you have learned something!

CPSIA information can be obtained
at www.ICGtesting.com
Printed in the USA
LVHW020930260521
688445LV00004B/472